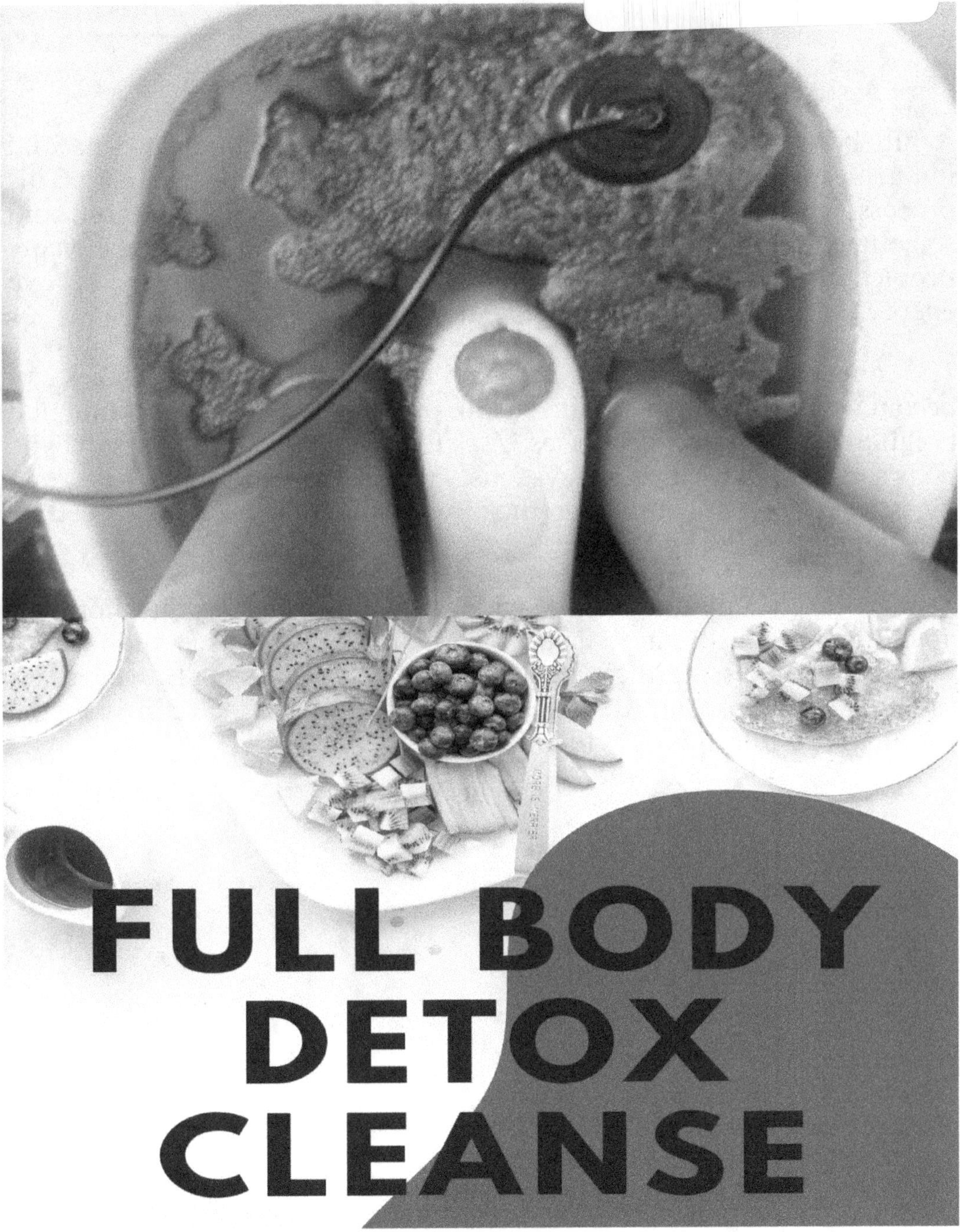

FULL BODY DETOX CLEANSE

INTRODUCTION

A full body detox cleanse is designed to help eliminate toxins and impurities from the body, promoting overall health and wellness. This process typically involves dietary changes, increased hydration, and sometimes the use of specific supplements or herbal remedies. Many people turn to detox cleanses to kickstart healthier habits, improve energy levels, and support digestive health.

The concept of detoxification is rooted in the belief that our bodies can become burdened with toxins from processed foods, environmental pollutants, and lifestyle choices. A detox cleanse aims to support the body's natural detoxification systems—primarily the liver, kidneys, and digestive tract—by providing them with the nutrients they need to function optimally.

While detox cleanses can vary widely in approach and duration, the goal remains consistent: to help individuals feel revitalized and foster a greater awareness of their health and dietary choices. However, it's essential to approach detoxing thoughtfully and to consider the potential benefits and risks involved.

TABLE OF CONTENTS

The term "detox" can refer to several concepts depending on the context:

1. **Medical Detoxification**: This involves the process of removing toxic substances from the body, often related to substance abuse treatment. Medical detox can be supervised by healthcare professionals and may involve medication to manage withdrawal symptoms.
2. **Dietary Detox**: This type of detox typically involves a specific diet or fasting regimen aimed at cleansing the body of toxins. These detox diets often include consuming juices, smoothies, or other natural foods believed to have detoxifying properties.
3. **Environmental Detox**: This refers to reducing exposure to environmental toxins, such as pollutants, chemicals, and heavy metals. This can involve lifestyle changes, using natural products, and avoiding certain materials or foods.
4. **Digital Detox**: This is a period during which a person refrains from using electronic devices such as smartphones and computers to reduce stress and focus on real-life interactions and activities.
5. **Emotional or Mental Detox**: This involves practices and activities aimed at reducing stress and negative emotions. It can include meditation, mindfulness, therapy, and other self-care practices.

Medical detoxification, often simply referred to as "detox," is the process of removing toxic substances from the body. This process is crucial in the treatment of individuals who have developed a dependence on substances such as alcohol, prescription medications, or illicit drugs. Here are some key aspects of medical detoxification:

Purpose

The primary goal of medical detoxification is to safely manage withdrawal symptoms when someone stops taking drugs or alcohol. Detox is usually the first step in a comprehensive addiction treatment plan.

Process

1. **Assessment:** A healthcare professional conducts a thorough evaluation to determine the individual's physical and mental health, the type and amount of substances used, and the presence of any co-occurring disorders.
2. **Stabilization:** This phase involves medical and psychological interventions to help the patient reach a stable, substance-free state. Medications may be prescribed to manage withdrawal symptoms and prevent complications.
3. **Transition to Treatment:** After stabilization, the patient is prepared for the next phase of treatment, which may include inpatient or outpatient rehabilitation, therapy, counseling, and support groups.

Withdrawal Symptoms

Withdrawal symptoms vary depending on the substance and the severity of the addiction. Common symptoms include:

- **Alcohol:** Anxiety, tremors, sweating, nausea, seizures, delirium tremens (DTs).
- **Opioids:** Muscle aches, agitation, insomnia, abdominal cramps, diarrhea.
- **Stimulants (e.g., cocaine, methamphetamine):** Fatigue, depression, increased appetite, disturbed sleep.

Medications Used in Detox

- **Alcohol:** Benzodiazepines (e.g., diazepam, lorazepam) to manage anxiety and seizures; vitamins (e.g., thiamine) to prevent Wernicke-Korsakoff syndrome.
- **Opioids:** Methadone, buprenorphine, or naltrexone to reduce cravings and withdrawal symptoms.
- **Benzodiazepines:** Gradual tapering of the drug to minimize withdrawal effects.

Safety Considerations

- **Medical Supervision**: Detox should be conducted under the supervision of healthcare professionals to ensure safety and effectiveness.
- **Individualized Care**: Treatment plans should be tailored to the individual's specific needs, considering factors such as the type of substance used, duration of use, and overall health.

Post-Detox Treatment

Detox is not a standalone treatment for addiction but rather the first step. Continued treatment is necessary to address the underlying causes of addiction and support long-term recovery. This may involve:

- **Therapy and Counseling**: Cognitive-behavioral therapy (CBT), motivational interviewing, and other therapeutic approaches.
- **Support Groups**: 12-step programs (e.g., Alcoholics Anonymous, Narcotics Anonymous) and other peer support groups.
- **Medication-Assisted Treatment (MAT)**: Ongoing use of medications to reduce the risk of relapse.

Dietary detox, or detox dieting, involves consuming specific foods and beverages to help remove toxins from the body and promote overall health. These detox diets are often short-term and focus on natural, whole foods. Here are key aspects of dietary detox:

Goals of Dietary Detox

- **Cleansing the Body**: Removing toxins that accumulate from food, the environment, and lifestyle choices.
- **Improving Digestion**: Enhancing the function of the digestive system.
- **Boosting Energy**: Increasing overall energy levels.
- **Supporting Weight Loss**: Promoting healthy weight loss through a nutrient-dense diet.

Common Components of Detox Diets

1. **Hydration**: Drinking plenty of water to help flush out toxins.
2. **Juices and Smoothies**: Consuming fresh fruit and vegetable juices or smoothies for vitamins, minerals, and antioxidants.
3. **Whole Foods**: Eating unprocessed foods, including fruits, vegetables, whole grains, nuts, and seeds.
4. **Herbal Teas**: Drinking herbal teas like green tea, dandelion tea, or ginger tea, which are believed to have detoxifying properties.
5. **Lemon Water**: Starting the day with lemon water to kickstart metabolism and digestion.
6. **Reducing Sugar and Processed Foods**: Avoiding added sugars, refined carbs, and processed foods.

Popular Detox Diets

1. **Juice Cleanses**: Consuming only fruit and vegetable juices for a few days.
2. **Smoothie Detox**: Replacing meals with nutrient-rich smoothies.
3. **Master Cleanse**: Drinking a mixture of lemon juice, maple syrup, cayenne pepper, and water.
4. **Raw Food Detox**: Eating only raw fruits, vegetables, nuts, and seeds.
5. **Liver Detox**: Consuming foods that support liver function, like leafy greens, beets, and garlic.

Benefits of Dietary Detox

- **Improved Digestion**: Increased fiber intake can promote better digestive health.
- **Increased Nutrient Intake**: Focusing on whole, natural foods can increase the intake of essential vitamins and minerals.
- **Reduced Inflammation**: Eliminating processed foods and sugars can reduce inflammation.
- **Weight Loss**: Some detox diets can help kickstart weight loss efforts.

Risks and Considerations

- **Nutritional Deficiencies**: Extreme detox diets may lack essential nutrients, leading to deficiencies.
- **Short-Term Focus**: Detox diets are not sustainable long-term solutions and may not lead to lasting health benefits.
- **Potential Side Effects**: Headaches, fatigue, and irritability can occur due to drastic dietary changes or calorie restriction.
- **Medical Conditions**: Individuals with certain health conditions or those taking medications should consult a healthcare professional before starting a detox diet.

Balanced Approach to Detox

For a more balanced and sustainable approach, consider integrating detoxifying principles into your regular diet:

- **Eat a Variety of Fruits and Vegetables**: Aim for a colorful plate to ensure a range of nutrients.
- **Stay Hydrated**: Drink plenty of water throughout the day.
- **Limit Processed Foods and Sugars**: Focus on whole, natural foods.
- **Incorporate Fiber-Rich Foods**: Include whole grains, legumes, and seeds to support digestion.
- **Practice Mindful Eating**: Pay attention to hunger and fullness cues, and choose nutrient-dense foods.

Environmental detox refers to reducing exposure to toxins in your surroundings to improve health and well-being. This type of detox focuses on minimizing contact with harmful chemicals, pollutants, and other environmental hazards. Here are key aspects and strategies for environmental detox:

Goals of Environmental Detox

- **Reducing Toxic Exposure**: Minimizing contact with harmful substances found in the environment.
- **Improving Indoor Air Quality**: Ensuring that the air you breathe indoors is clean and free from pollutants.

- **Promoting a Healthier Home Environment**: Creating a living space that supports overall health and well-being.

Common Environmental Toxins

1. **Air Pollutants**: Smoke, pollen, mold, pet dander, and chemicals from household cleaners.
2. **Water Contaminants**: Heavy metals, chlorine, pesticides, and industrial pollutants.
3. **Household Chemicals**: Cleaning products, pesticides, and personal care items containing harmful ingredients.
4. **Plastics**: Bisphenol A (BPA) and phthalates found in plastic containers and packaging.
5. **Heavy Metals**: Lead, mercury, and cadmium from various sources, including paint, plumbing, and certain foods.

Strategies for Environmental Detox

1. Improving Indoor Air Quality

- **Ventilation**: Ensure proper ventilation in your home by opening windows and using exhaust fans.
- **Air Purifiers**: Use air purifiers with HEPA filters to remove airborne particles and pollutants.
- **Houseplants**: Add indoor plants that can help purify the air, such as spider plants, snake plants, and peace lilies.
- **Regular Cleaning**: Vacuum and dust regularly to reduce allergens and dust mites.
- **Avoid Smoking Indoors**: Keep indoor air smoke-free to prevent exposure to harmful chemicals.

2. Drinking Clean Water

- **Water Filters**: Use water filters to remove contaminants from tap water. Options include activated carbon filters, reverse osmosis systems, and pitcher filters.
- **Avoid Plastic Bottles**: Use glass or stainless steel water bottles to avoid chemicals leaching from plastic.

3. Choosing Safer Household Products

- **Natural Cleaning Products**: Use cleaning products made from natural ingredients like vinegar, baking soda, and essential oils.
- **Non-Toxic Personal Care Products**: Opt for personal care products free from parabens, sulfates, and synthetic fragrances.
- **Avoid Pesticides**: Use natural pest control methods, such as diatomaceous earth, essential oils, and traps.

4. Reducing Plastic Use

- **Glass and Stainless Steel Containers**: Store food and beverages in glass or stainless steel containers instead of plastic.
- **Avoid Heating Plastics**: Do not microwave food in plastic containers, as heat can cause chemicals to leach into the food.
- **Reusable Bags and Wraps**: Use reusable cloth bags and beeswax wraps instead of plastic bags and wraps.

5. Minimizing Heavy Metal Exposure

- **Lead-Safe Practices**: If you live in an older home, ensure that lead-based paint is properly sealed or removed by professionals.
- **Avoid Mercury**: Be cautious with certain seafood that may contain high levels of mercury, such as shark, swordfish, and king mackerel.
- **Safe Electronics Disposal**: Properly dispose of electronic waste to prevent heavy metals from leaching into the environment.

Additional Tips for Environmental Detox

- **Green Building Materials**: When renovating or building, choose materials with low or no volatile organic compounds (VOCs).
- **Natural Textiles**: Use organic cotton, wool, and other natural fibers for clothing, bedding, and upholstery.
- **Regularly Check for Mold**: Inspect your home for mold and take steps to remediate it promptly if found.

Benefits of Environmental Detox

- **Improved Respiratory Health**: Reduced exposure to air pollutants can improve lung function and decrease respiratory issues.
- **Enhanced Overall Health**: Lowering exposure to harmful chemicals can decrease the risk of various health problems, including hormonal imbalances and certain cancers.
- **Better Indoor Living Environment**: Creating a cleaner and safer home environment promotes overall well-being and comfort.

A digital detox involves taking a break from electronic devices like smartphones, computers, tablets, and social media platforms to reduce stress and improve overall well-being. Here are key aspects of a digital detox:

Goals of a Digital Detox

- **Reducing Screen Time**: Decreasing the amount of time spent on electronic devices.
- **Improving Mental Health**: Reducing anxiety, stress, and feelings of overwhelm associated with constant connectivity.
- **Enhancing Focus and Productivity**: Minimizing distractions to improve concentration and efficiency.
- **Promoting Real-Life Interactions**: Encouraging more face-to-face social interactions and activities.

Signs You Might Need a Digital Detox

- Feeling overwhelmed or stressed by constant notifications and online interactions.
- Experiencing difficulty concentrating or completing tasks due to frequent digital distractions.
- Noticing a negative impact on relationships due to excessive screen time.
- Feeling anxious or depressed after using social media.
- Having trouble sleeping due to screen use before bed.

Steps for a Successful Digital Detox

1. Set Clear Goals

- Define what you want to achieve with your digital detox, such as reduced stress, better sleep, or more time for hobbies.

2. Establish Boundaries

- Decide on specific times of day when you will avoid using electronic devices, such as during meals or before bedtime.
- Create tech-free zones in your home, like the bedroom or dining area.

3. Plan Alternative Activities

- Engage in activities that don't involve screens, such as reading, exercising, cooking, or spending time outdoors.
- Take up a new hobby or revisit an old one to fill the time you would normally spend on devices.

4. Inform Others

- Let friends, family, and colleagues know about your digital detox to manage their expectations regarding your availability.

5. Use Technology to Help

- Utilize apps that track and limit screen time, block distracting websites, or remind you to take breaks from your device.
- Adjust settings on your phone or computer to reduce notifications and alerts.

6. Gradual Reduction

- If a complete break feels too challenging, start by gradually reducing your screen time each day until you reach your desired level.

Tips for Maintaining a Digital Detox

1. Monitor Your Usage

- Keep track of your screen time and identify patterns that may need adjustment.
- Reflect on how you feel after reducing your digital use and make necessary changes.

2. Practice Mindfulness

- Be mindful of your digital habits and make conscious decisions about when and how to use technology.
- Use mindfulness techniques, such as meditation or deep breathing, to manage the urge to check your devices.

3. Stay Accountable

- Share your goals with a friend or family member who can help keep you accountable.
- Join a group or community that supports digital detox efforts.

Benefits of a Digital Detox

- **Improved Mental Health**: Reduced anxiety, stress, and feelings of overwhelm from constant connectivity.
- **Better Sleep**: Enhanced sleep quality by reducing screen use before bedtime.
- **Increased Productivity**: Improved focus and concentration by minimizing digital distractions.
- **Enhanced Relationships**: More meaningful interactions with loved ones by being present and attentive.
- **Greater Sense of Well-Being**: Increased engagement in real-life activities and hobbies.

Challenges and Solutions

- **Boredom**: Find engaging activities to fill the time usually spent on devices.

- **FOMO (Fear of Missing Out)**: Remind yourself of the benefits and focus on enjoying the present moment.
- **Work Requirements**: If your job requires screen time, set boundaries for non-work hours and take regular breaks.

An emotional and mental detox involves taking steps to clear your mind and heart of negative thoughts, emotions, and stress. This type of detox can improve mental clarity, emotional balance, and overall well-being. Here are key aspects and strategies for an emotional and mental detox:

Goals of Emotional and Mental Detox

- **Reducing Stress**: Decreasing levels of stress and anxiety.
- **Improving Emotional Health**: Letting go of negative emotions such as anger, resentment, and sadness.
- **Enhancing Mental Clarity**: Clearing mental clutter to improve focus and decision-making.
- **Promoting Positive Thinking**: Cultivating a more positive and resilient mindset.

Signs You Might Need an Emotional and Mental Detox

- Feeling overwhelmed by emotions or stress.
- Struggling with persistent negative thoughts or a critical inner voice.
- Experiencing difficulty concentrating or making decisions.
- Noticing a decline in overall happiness and satisfaction with life.
- Feeling emotionally drained or burnt out.

Steps for an Effective Emotional and Mental Detox

1. Practice Mindfulness and Meditation

- **Mindfulness**: Engage in mindfulness practices to stay present and aware of your thoughts and feelings without judgment. This can help reduce stress and increase emotional resilience.
- **Meditation**: Set aside time each day for meditation to quiet the mind, reduce anxiety, and improve emotional well-being.

Techniques like deep breathing, guided imagery, and body scanning can be particularly helpful.

2. Journaling

- **Express Your Thoughts and Emotions**: Write down your thoughts and feelings to gain insight and release pent-up emotions.
- **Gratitude Journaling**: Keep a gratitude journal to focus on positive aspects of your life, which can help shift your mindset and improve mood.

3. Practice Self-Care

- **Physical Activity**: Engage in regular exercise to reduce stress and improve mood. Activities like yoga, walking, or dancing can be particularly beneficial.
- **Relaxation Techniques**: Incorporate relaxation techniques such as deep breathing, progressive muscle relaxation, or aromatherapy into your routine.

4. Limit Negative Influences

- **Media Consumption**: Reduce exposure to negative news, social media, and other sources of stress or negativity.
- **Toxic Relationships**: Identify and limit interactions with people who consistently bring negativity or drain your energy.

5. Cultivate Positive Relationships

- **Social Support**: Spend time with supportive friends and family who uplift and encourage you.
- **Positive Communication**: Practice open and positive communication to strengthen relationships and resolve conflicts.

6. Set Boundaries

- **Personal Boundaries**: Establish and maintain boundaries to protect your emotional well-being. Learn to say no to commitments that cause unnecessary stress.

- **Digital Boundaries**: Limit time spent on digital devices and social media to prevent information overload and reduce stress.

Additional Strategies for Emotional and Mental Detox

1. Engage in Creative Activities

- **Art and Music**: Participate in creative activities like painting, drawing, or playing a musical instrument to express emotions and reduce stress.
- **Hobbies**: Revisit old hobbies or take up new ones that bring joy and relaxation.

2. Practice Positive Affirmations

- **Affirmations**: Use positive affirmations to challenge and replace negative thoughts. Repeat affirmations daily to reinforce a positive mindset.

3. Seek Professional Help

- **Therapy and Counseling**: Consider speaking with a therapist or counselor to work through emotional issues and develop coping strategies.
- **Support Groups**: Join support groups to connect with others facing similar challenges and share experiences.

Benefits of Emotional and Mental Detox

- **Reduced Stress and Anxiety**: Lower levels of stress and anxiety, leading to improved mental health.
- **Improved Emotional Balance**: Greater ability to manage emotions and respond to challenges with resilience.
- **Enhanced Mental Clarity**: Better focus, concentration, and decision-making.
- **Increased Positivity**: A more positive outlook on life and improved overall well-being.

Challenges and Solutions

- **Consistency**: Maintaining new habits can be challenging. Set realistic goals and be patient with yourself.
- **Overcoming Resistance**: It's normal to feel resistance to change. Focus on the benefits and take small, manageable steps.
- **Seeking Support**: Don't hesitate to seek support from friends, family, or professionals if you need help.

Detox smoothies can be a delicious and nutritious way to support your body's natural detoxification processes. Here are some recipes for detox smoothies, each designed to provide a variety of vitamins, minerals, and antioxidants to help cleanse your system and boost your overall health.

1. Green Detox Smoothie

Ingredients:

- 1 cup spinach
- 1 cup kale
- 1 banana
- 1 apple, cored and chopped
- 1/2 cucumber
- 1 lemon, juiced
- 1 tablespoon chia seeds
- 1 cup water or coconut water

Instructions:

1. Add all ingredients to a blender.
2. Blend until smooth.
3. Add more water if needed to reach your desired consistency.

2. Berry Detox Smoothie

Ingredients:

- 1 cup mixed berries (strawberries, blueberries, raspberries)
- 1/2 banana

- 1 tablespoon flaxseeds
- 1 cup unsweetened almond milk
- 1 tablespoon honey or maple syrup (optional)
- A handful of spinach (optional)

Instructions:

1. Add all ingredients to a blender.
2. Blend until smooth.
3. Add ice cubes if you prefer a colder smoothie.

3. Tropical Detox Smoothie

Ingredients:

- 1 cup pineapple chunks
- 1/2 cup mango chunks
- 1 banana
- 1/2 cup coconut water
- 1/2 teaspoon turmeric powder
- 1/2 teaspoon grated ginger
- A handful of fresh mint leaves

Instructions:

1. Add all ingredients to a blender.
2. Blend until smooth.
3. Serve immediately.

4. Citrus Detox Smoothie

Ingredients:

- 1 orange, peeled and segmented
- 1/2 grapefruit, peeled and segmented
- 1/2 lemon, juiced
- 1/2 cup carrots, chopped
- 1/2 cup Greek yogurt
- 1 tablespoon flaxseed oil
- 1 cup water or coconut water

Instructions:

1. Add all ingredients to a blender.
2. Blend until smooth.
3. Add ice cubes if desired.

5. Beet Detox Smoothie

Ingredients:

- 1 small beet, peeled and chopped
- 1 apple, cored and chopped
- 1 carrot, chopped
- 1/2 inch fresh ginger, peeled and chopped
- 1 tablespoon chia seeds
- 1 cup water or coconut water

Instructions:

1. Add all ingredients to a blender.
2. Blend until smooth.
3. Strain through a fine-mesh sieve if you prefer a smoother texture.

6. Avocado Detox Smoothie

Ingredients:

- 1/2 avocado
- 1 banana
- 1 cup spinach
- 1 cup unsweetened almond milk
- 1 tablespoon hemp seeds
- 1/2 teaspoon spirulina powder (optional)
- 1/2 teaspoon matcha powder (optional)

Instructions:

1. Add all ingredients to a blender.
2. Blend until smooth.
3. Adjust consistency with more almond milk if needed.

7. Refreshing Cucumber Mint Smoothie

Ingredients:

- 1 cucumber, peeled and chopped
- 1 green apple, cored and chopped
- 1/2 cup fresh mint leaves
- 1/2 lemon, juiced
- 1/2 cup water or coconut water
- Ice cubes (optional)

Instructions:

1. Add all ingredients to a blender.
2. Blend until smooth.
3. Serve chilled.

Tips for Making Detox Smoothies

- **Organic Ingredients:** Whenever possible, use organic fruits and vegetables to avoid pesticides and other chemicals.
- **Freshness:** Consume your smoothies immediately after preparation to retain maximum nutrients.
- **Variety:** Experiment with different fruits, vegetables, and superfoods to keep your smoothies exciting and nutritionally balanced.
- **Hydration:** Adding coconut water or water helps in maintaining hydration and improving the texture of the smoothie.

Detox Soups

1. Cleansing Green Soup

Ingredients:

- 1 tablespoon olive oil
- 1 onion, chopped
- 2 cloves garlic, minced
- 4 cups vegetable broth
- 2 cups kale, chopped

- 2 cups spinach
- 1 zucchini, chopped
- 1 cup broccoli florets
- 1 cup peas
- 1 lemon, juiced
- Salt and pepper to taste

Instructions:

1. Heat olive oil in a large pot over medium heat.
2. Add onion and garlic, sauté until translucent.
3. Add vegetable broth, kale, spinach, zucchini, and broccoli. Bring to a boil.
4. Reduce heat and simmer for 15-20 minutes until vegetables are tender.
5. Add peas and cook for another 5 minutes.
6. Remove from heat and let cool slightly.
7. Blend the soup until smooth using an immersion blender or in batches in a regular blender.
8. Stir in lemon juice, and season with salt and pepper.

2. Carrot Ginger Detox Soup

Ingredients:

- 1 tablespoon coconut oil
- 1 onion, chopped
- 2 cloves garlic, minced
- 1 tablespoon fresh ginger, grated
- 6 large carrots, peeled and chopped
- 4 cups vegetable broth
- 1 cup coconut milk
- Salt and pepper to taste
- Fresh cilantro for garnish

Instructions:

1. Heat coconut oil in a large pot over medium heat.
2. Add onion, garlic, and ginger, and sauté until fragrant.

3. Add carrots and vegetable broth. Bring to a boil.
4. Reduce heat and simmer for 20 minutes until carrots are tender.
5. Blend the soup until smooth using an immersion blender or in batches in a regular blender.
6. Stir in coconut milk and season with salt and pepper.
7. Garnish with fresh cilantro.

Detox Salads

1. Kale and Quinoa Detox Salad

Ingredients:

- 2 cups kale, chopped
- 1 cup cooked quinoa
- 1/2 cup shredded carrots
- 1/2 cup red cabbage, thinly sliced
- 1/4 cup pumpkin seeds
- 1 avocado, diced
- 1/4 cup dried cranberries
- 1/4 cup fresh lemon juice
- 2 tablespoons olive oil
- Salt and pepper to taste

Instructions:

1. In a large bowl, massage kale with lemon juice and a pinch of salt until softened.
2. Add cooked quinoa, shredded carrots, red cabbage, pumpkin seeds, avocado, and dried cranberries.
3. Drizzle with olive oil and season with salt and pepper.
4. Toss to combine and serve.

2. Detox Beet Salad

Ingredients:

- 2 medium beets, roasted and diced
- 1 apple, diced

- 1/4 cup walnuts, chopped
- 1/4 cup goat cheese, crumbled (optional)
- 2 tablespoons fresh parsley, chopped
- 2 tablespoons balsamic vinegar
- 1 tablespoon olive oil
- Salt and pepper to taste

Instructions:

1. In a large bowl, combine roasted beets, apple, walnuts, goat cheese, and parsley.
2. In a small bowl, whisk together balsamic vinegar, olive oil, salt, and pepper.
3. Pour the dressing over the salad and toss to combine.

Detox Teas

1. Ginger Turmeric Detox Tea

Ingredients:

- 2 cups water
- 1-inch piece fresh ginger, sliced
- 1/2 teaspoon ground turmeric (or 1-inch fresh turmeric root, sliced)
- 1 tablespoon honey
- 1 lemon, juiced

Instructions:

1. In a small pot, bring water to a boil.
2. Add ginger and turmeric, reduce heat, and simmer for 10 minutes.
3. Strain the tea into a cup.
4. Stir in honey and lemon juice.
5. Enjoy warm.

2. Dandelion Detox Tea

Ingredients:

- 1 teaspoon dried dandelion root
- 1 teaspoon dried dandelion leaf
- 2 cups water
- 1 teaspoon honey (optional)
- Lemon wedge (optional)

Instructions:

1. In a small pot, bring water to a boil.
2. Add dandelion root and leaf, reduce heat, and simmer for 10-15 minutes.
3. Strain the tea into a cup.
4. Sweeten with honey and add a lemon wedge if desired.
5. Enjoy warm.

Detox Infused Waters

1. Lemon Cucumber Mint Water

Ingredients:

- 1 lemon, sliced
- 1/2 cucumber, sliced
- A handful of fresh mint leaves
- 1 quart water

Instructions:

1. Add lemon slices, cucumber slices, and mint leaves to a pitcher.
2. Fill with water and let infuse in the refrigerator for at least 1 hour before serving.

2. Berry Detox Water

Ingredients:

- 1/2 cup strawberries, sliced
- 1/2 cup blueberries
- 1/2 cup raspberries
- 1 quart water

Instructions:

1. Add strawberries, blueberries, and raspberries to a pitcher.
2. Fill with water and let infuse in the refrigerator for at least 1 hour before serving.

A thorough assessment for medical detoxification is essential to ensure a safe and effective detox process, especially for individuals withdrawing from substances such as alcohol, opioids, benzodiazepines, and other drugs. This assessment typically involves evaluating the patient's physical, psychological, and social health to determine the appropriate level of care and interventions needed. Here's a comprehensive guide to the components of a medical detox assessment:

1. Medical History and Physical Examination

- **Substance Use History:** Detailed information about the types, amounts, duration, and patterns of substance use.
- **Previous Detox Attempts:** History of past detoxifications, including any complications or relapses.
- **Medical Conditions:** Identification of chronic and acute medical conditions that may affect the detox process.
- **Medications:** Current medications, including over-the-counter drugs and supplements.
- **Allergies:** Known drug or food allergies.
- **Physical Examination:** Comprehensive physical exam to identify any immediate health concerns or complications related to substance use.

2. Psychological Assessment

- **Mental Health History**: Evaluation of past and present mental health conditions, including depression, anxiety, bipolar disorder, schizophrenia, etc.
- **Current Mental Status**: Assessment of current mood, thought processes, cognitive function, and risk of self-harm or harm to others.
- **Behavioral Health**: Patterns of behavior related to substance use, including triggers and coping mechanisms.

3. Substance-Specific Assessment

- **Withdrawal Symptoms**: Identification and assessment of withdrawal symptoms, including their severity and frequency.
- **Risk of Complications**: Evaluation of potential risks associated with withdrawal from specific substances, such as delirium tremens (DTs) in alcohol withdrawal or seizures in benzodiazepine withdrawal.
- **Screening Tools**: Utilization of standardized tools to assess withdrawal symptoms, such as the Clinical Institute Withdrawal Assessment for Alcohol (CIWA-Ar) or Clinical Opiate Withdrawal Scale (COWS).

4. Laboratory Tests

- **Blood Tests**: Comprehensive metabolic panel, liver function tests, complete blood count, and tests for infectious diseases (e.g., HIV, hepatitis).
- **Urine Drug Screen**: Identification of substances currently in the patient's system.
- **Other Tests**: As needed, based on individual health status (e.g., ECG for cardiovascular assessment).

5. Social Assessment

- **Support System**: Evaluation of the patient's support system, including family, friends, and social networks.

- **Living Situation**: Assessment of the patient's living environment and its impact on their recovery process.
- **Employment and Financial Status**: Understanding of employment status and financial stability.
- **Legal Issues**: Identification of any legal issues related to substance use.

6. Treatment Planning

- **Level of Care**: Determination of the appropriate level of care based on the assessment findings (e.g., inpatient detox, outpatient detox, medically supervised detox).
- **Intervention Strategies**: Development of a personalized treatment plan, including medication management, counseling, and support services.
- **Safety Planning**: Creation of a safety plan to address any immediate risks, such as suicidal ideation or potential for withdrawal complications.

7. Follow-Up and Aftercare

- **Continuity of Care**: Planning for ongoing care post-detox, including referrals to addiction treatment programs, mental health services, and support groups.
- **Relapse Prevention**: Strategies to prevent relapse, including education on coping skills, triggers, and ongoing support.

Key Considerations for Medical Detox Assessment

- **Confidentiality**: Ensuring patient confidentiality throughout the assessment process.
- **Patient-Centered Approach**: Involving the patient in the assessment and treatment planning process to address their unique needs and preferences.
- **Multidisciplinary Team**: Collaboration with a team of healthcare professionals, including doctors, nurses, mental health specialists, and social workers, to provide comprehensive care.

Stabilization in medical detoxification is a critical phase that involves managing acute withdrawal symptoms and stabilizing the patient's physical and psychological health. The goal is to ensure the patient's safety, comfort, and readiness for further treatment. Here are the key components and considerations for stabilization in medical detox:

1. Initial Assessment and Monitoring

- **Comprehensive Assessment**: Conduct a thorough initial assessment to understand the patient's medical history, substance use history, and current condition.
- **Continuous Monitoring**: Regularly monitor vital signs, withdrawal symptoms, and overall health status to detect and manage any complications promptly. Use standardized tools like CIWA-Ar for alcohol withdrawal and COWS for opioid withdrawal.

2. Medical Interventions

- **Medication Management**: Administer medications to alleviate withdrawal symptoms and prevent complications. Commonly used medications include:
    - **Benzodiazepines**: For managing alcohol withdrawal symptoms and preventing seizures.
    - **Methadone or Buprenorphine**: For opioid withdrawal management.
    - **Clonidine**: To alleviate symptoms of opioid withdrawal.
    - **Antipsychotics or Antidepressants**: If indicated for co-occurring mental health conditions.
- **Hydration and Nutrition**: Ensure adequate hydration and nutritional support to address any deficiencies and support overall health.

3. Symptom Management

- **Pain and Discomfort**: Use appropriate analgesics and comfort measures to manage pain and discomfort.
- **Sleep Disturbances**: Address sleep issues with non-addictive sleep aids or behavioral interventions.

- **Nausea and Vomiting**: Administer antiemetics to control nausea and vomiting.

4. Psychological Support

- **Emotional Support**: Provide reassurance and emotional support to help the patient cope with anxiety, fear, or other emotional challenges during detox.
- **Counseling**: Offer brief counseling sessions to address immediate psychological needs and motivate the patient for further treatment.

5. Safety and Risk Management

- **Seizure Precautions**: Implement seizure precautions for patients at risk, such as those undergoing alcohol or benzodiazepine withdrawal.
- **Fall Precautions**: Ensure a safe environment to prevent falls, especially for patients experiencing dizziness or confusion.
- **Suicide Risk Assessment**: Regularly assess the risk of suicide and take appropriate measures to ensure patient safety.

6. Communication and Education

- **Patient Education**: Educate the patient about the detox process, withdrawal symptoms, and the importance of stabilization.
- **Family Involvement**: Involve family members or significant others in the process, if appropriate, to provide additional support and information.

7. Preparing for Transition to Further Treatment

- **Aftercare Planning**: Begin planning for the next phase of treatment, whether it's inpatient rehabilitation, outpatient therapy, or another form of ongoing care.
- **Referral and Coordination**: Coordinate with addiction treatment providers, mental health professionals, and other support services to ensure a smooth transition.

Common Challenges and Solutions in Stabilization

- **Severe Withdrawal Symptoms**: Manage severe symptoms with appropriate medications and close monitoring. Adjust treatment plans as needed.
- **Co-Occurring Disorders**: Address co-occurring mental health disorders with integrated treatment approaches, involving specialists as necessary.
- **Patient Reluctance**: Engage patients in motivational interviewing to increase their willingness to participate in ongoing treatment.

Case Example: Alcohol Detox Stabilization

1. **Assessment**: A patient presents with severe alcohol withdrawal symptoms, including tremors, sweating, and anxiety.
2. **Medication Management**: Administer a benzodiazepine like diazepam to manage withdrawal symptoms and prevent seizures.
3. **Monitoring**: Regularly check vital signs and use CIWA-Ar to assess withdrawal severity.
4. **Support**: Provide emotional support and educate the patient about the importance of stabilization and the next steps in treatment.
5. **Aftercare**: Plan for the patient's transition to an inpatient rehabilitation program for continued care and recovery support.

Key Points to Remember

- **Safety First**: Prioritize patient safety through careful monitoring and appropriate interventions.
- **Comprehensive Care**: Address both physical and psychological aspects of withdrawal.
- **Patient-Centered Approach**: Involve the patient in their care and provide support and education throughout the process.
- **Preparation for Next Steps**: Ensure the patient is ready and has a clear plan for continued treatment after stabilization.

Withdrawal symptoms can vary widely depending on the substance involved and the individual's overall health. Here's an overview of withdrawal symptoms associated with common substances typically requiring medical detox:

1. Alcohol Withdrawal Symptoms

- **Mild Symptoms**: Anxiety, insomnia, nausea, sweating, tremors, headaches.
- **Moderate Symptoms**: Increased heart rate, elevated blood pressure, hallucinations (visual or auditory).
- **Severe Symptoms**: Delirium tremens (DTs) characterized by severe confusion, agitation, seizures, and severe autonomic instability.

2. Opioid Withdrawal Symptoms

- **Early Symptoms** (within hours): Anxiety, muscle aches, insomnia, sweating, runny nose, teary eyes.
- **Later Symptoms** (1-3 days): Nausea, vomiting, diarrhea, abdominal cramps, goosebumps, dilated pupils.
- **Duration**: Symptoms can last from a few days to several weeks, depending on the opioid and duration of use.

3. Benzodiazepine Withdrawal Symptoms

- **Mild Symptoms**: Anxiety, insomnia, irritability, restlessness.
- **Moderate Symptoms**: Increased heart rate, muscle spasms, dizziness, and difficulty concentrating.
- **Severe Symptoms**: Seizures, hallucinations, delirium, and life-threatening complications.

4. Stimulant Withdrawal Symptoms (e.g., cocaine, methamphetamine)

- **Symptoms**: Fatigue, increased appetite, depression, anxiety, agitation, vivid and unpleasant dreams, and cravings.
- **Duration**: Symptoms can last from a few days to several weeks, depending on the substance and usage patterns.

5. Cannabis Withdrawal Symptoms

- **Symptoms**: Irritability, insomnia, decreased appetite, anxiety, mood swings, and cravings.

- **Duration**: Symptoms typically peak within the first week and can last up to two weeks.

6. Nicotine Withdrawal Symptoms

- **Symptoms**: Irritability, anxiety, difficulty concentrating, increased appetite, cravings, and sleep disturbances.
- **Duration**: Symptoms can last several weeks, with cravings often persisting for months.

Management Strategies

- **Medication**: Use of specific medications to alleviate withdrawal symptoms, such as benzodiazepines for alcohol withdrawal or methadone/buprenorphine for opioid withdrawal.
- **Supportive Care**: Providing emotional support and counseling, hydration, nutrition, and managing comorbid conditions.
- **Monitoring**: Close monitoring for severe symptoms, especially with alcohol and benzodiazepine withdrawal, to prevent complications.

Medications used in detoxification aim to alleviate withdrawal symptoms, reduce cravings, and ensure patient safety. Here's a breakdown of common medications used for detox from various substances:

1. Alcohol Detox

- **Benzodiazepines:**
    - **Examples**: Diazepam (Valium), Lorazepam (Ativan), Chlordiazepoxide (Librium).
    - **Purpose**: Reduce withdrawal symptoms and prevent seizures.
- **Adjunct Medications:**
    - **Gabapentin**: May help with anxiety and insomnia.
    - **Clonidine**: Can reduce autonomic symptoms (sweating, rapid heartbeat).

2. Opioid Detox

- **Methadone:**
  - **Purpose:** A long-acting opioid used to ease withdrawal symptoms and cravings.
- **Buprenorphine:**
  - **Purpose:** Partial opioid agonist that helps manage withdrawal and reduces cravings.
- **Naltrexone:**
  - **Purpose:** An opioid antagonist that blocks the effects of opioids; used after detox to prevent relapse.
- **Clonidine:**
  - **Purpose:** Can alleviate withdrawal symptoms like anxiety and agitation.

3. Benzodiazepine Detox

- **Tapering with Long-Acting Benzodiazepines:**
  - **Examples:** Diazepam or Chlordiazepoxide.
  - **Purpose:** Gradual reduction to minimize withdrawal symptoms.
- **Adjunct Medications:**
  - **Antidepressants or Antipsychotics:** May be used for co-occurring mood disorders or severe anxiety.

4. Stimulant Detox (e.g., cocaine, methamphetamine)

- **No specific medications:**
  - Treatment is primarily supportive, focusing on managing symptoms (e.g., anxiety, depression) and providing behavioral therapies.

5. Nicotine Detox

- **Nicotine Replacement Therapy (NRT):**
  - **Examples:** Nicotine patches, gum, lozenges.
  - **Purpose:** Reduces withdrawal symptoms and cravings.
- **Bupropion (Zyban):**

- Purpose: An antidepressant that helps reduce cravings and withdrawal symptoms.
- **Varenicline (Chantix)**:
  - **Purpose**: Reduces withdrawal symptoms and cravings by acting on nicotine receptors.

General Considerations

- **Individualized Treatment**: Medication regimens should be tailored to the individual's specific substance use history, withdrawal severity, and any co-occurring mental health conditions.
- **Monitoring**: Patients should be closely monitored for side effects and withdrawal symptom management throughout the detox process.
- **Multidisciplinary Approach**: Combining medication with counseling and behavioral therapies improves treatment outcomes.

Safety considerations in medical detoxification are critical to ensure the well-being of patients as they undergo withdrawal from substances. Here are key safety considerations:

1. Comprehensive Assessment

- **Initial Evaluation**: Conduct thorough assessments of medical, psychological, and substance use history to identify potential complications.
- **Withdrawal Severity**: Utilize standardized assessment tools (e.g., CIWA-Ar for alcohol, COWS for opioids) to evaluate withdrawal severity and risks.

2. Monitoring

- **Vital Signs**: Regularly monitor blood pressure, heart rate, respiratory rate, and temperature to detect any abnormalities.
- **Withdrawal Symptoms**: Continuously assess and document withdrawal symptoms to adjust treatment as necessary.

- **Mental Status**: Monitor for changes in mental status, especially for signs of severe anxiety, agitation, or hallucinations.

3. Medical Interventions

- **Seizure Precautions**: Implement precautions for patients at risk of seizures, particularly those withdrawing from alcohol or benzodiazepines.
- **Emergency Protocols**: Establish protocols for managing emergencies, including seizures, severe agitation, or delirium tremens (DTs).

4. Medication Management

- **Appropriate Use of Medications**: Use medications to manage withdrawal symptoms and prevent complications, ensuring dosing is tailored to the individual.
- **Avoidance of Polypharmacy**: Minimize the use of multiple medications that could lead to interactions or increased side effects.

5. Supportive Care

- **Hydration and Nutrition**: Ensure proper hydration and nutrition to support the patient's physical health during detox.
- **Comfort Measures**: Provide non-pharmacological interventions (e.g., warm blankets, calm environment) to enhance comfort.

6. Mental Health Considerations

- **Suicide Risk Assessment**: Regularly assess and address the risk of self-harm or suicide, particularly in individuals with a history of mental health disorders.
- **Psychological Support**: Offer counseling or supportive therapy to help manage anxiety and emotional distress during detox.

7. Environment

- **Safe Setting**: Ensure that the detox environment is secure and supportive, minimizing potential triggers for substance use.

- **Supervision**: Maintain appropriate levels of supervision based on the severity of withdrawal and risk factors.

8. Transition Planning

- **Aftercare Coordination**: Plan for a smooth transition to ongoing treatment post-detox, including referrals to rehabilitation programs and support groups.
- **Relapse Prevention**: Provide education on recognizing triggers and coping strategies to prevent relapse.

9. Staff Training

- **Education**: Ensure that staff are trained in recognizing and managing withdrawal symptoms, understanding detox protocols, and responding to medical emergencies.

10. Family Involvement

- **Support Systems**: Engage family members in the process, providing education and support to help them understand the detox process and recovery journey.

By implementing these safety considerations, healthcare providers can create a supportive environment that enhances patient safety and promotes successful detoxification.

Post-detox treatment is crucial for sustaining recovery after the initial detoxification process. It focuses on addressing the psychological, social, and behavioral aspects of addiction. Here are key components of post-detox treatment:

1. Continuing Care

- **Rehabilitation Programs**: Transition to inpatient or outpatient rehab programs that provide structured support and therapeutic interventions.
- **Counseling and Therapy**: Engage in individual therapy (e.g., cognitive-behavioral therapy) and group therapy to address underlying issues and develop coping strategies.

2. Relapse Prevention

- **Education**: Learn about triggers and warning signs of relapse, and develop personalized relapse prevention plans.
- **Coping Strategies**: Develop skills for managing cravings, stress, and difficult emotions without resorting to substance use.

3. Support Groups

- **12-Step Programs**: Participate in support groups like Alcoholics Anonymous (AA) or Narcotics Anonymous (NA) for peer support and accountability.
- **Sober Living Environments**: Consider living in sober housing to provide a supportive and substance-free environment during early recovery.

4. Medication-Assisted Treatment (MAT)

- **Ongoing Medication**: If applicable, continue medications like naltrexone, buprenorphine, or methadone to manage cravings and reduce the risk of relapse.

5. Holistic Approaches

- **Wellness Practices**: Incorporate holistic practices such as yoga, mindfulness, meditation, and exercise to promote overall well-being.
- **Nutritional Support**: Focus on a balanced diet to support physical recovery and mental health.

6. Family Involvement

- **Family Therapy**: Engage family members in therapy to address dynamics that may impact recovery and to rebuild relationships.
- **Education**: Provide education for family members about addiction and recovery to foster a supportive home environment.

7. Ongoing Monitoring and Support

- **Regular Check-Ins**: Schedule follow-up appointments with healthcare providers to monitor progress and address any challenges.
- **Crisis Management**: Have a plan in place for managing potential crises or relapse triggers.

8. Lifestyle Changes

- **Building a Supportive Network**: Surround oneself with positive influences and a supportive community.
- **Developing New Interests**: Encourage exploration of new hobbies and interests to create a fulfilling and substance-free life.

9. Employment and Education Support

- **Job Training and Support**: Access resources for job training, educational opportunities, and career counseling.
- **Skill Development**: Focus on developing life skills that support independence and stability.

10. Long-Term Planning

- **Setting Goals**: Establish personal goals for recovery, including health, relationships, and career aspirations.
- **Maintaining Motivation**: Regularly review and adjust goals to maintain motivation and commitment to recovery.

By following a comprehensive post-detox treatment plan, individuals can enhance their chances of sustained recovery and build a fulfilling life free from substance use.

The goals of dietary detox can vary based on individual needs and preferences, but generally, they focus on promoting overall health and well-being. Here are the main goals of dietary detox:

1. Elimination of Toxins

- **Reduce Toxic Load**: Aim to eliminate or reduce exposure to toxins from processed foods, additives, and environmental sources.
- **Support Liver Function**: Enhance liver health, which plays a key role in detoxification.

2. Improved Digestion

- **Gut Health**: Promote a healthy gut microbiome through the intake of fiber-rich foods and probiotics.
- **Reduce Inflammation**: Identify and eliminate foods that may cause digestive discomfort or inflammation.

3. Weight Management

- **Promote Healthy Eating Habits**: Encourage the consumption of whole, nutrient-dense foods to support weight loss or maintenance.
- **Balanced Nutrition**: Foster an awareness of portion control and balanced macronutrient intake.

4. Increased Energy Levels

- **Boost Vitality**: Enhance overall energy levels through improved nutrition and the elimination of energy-draining foods.
- **Stable Blood Sugar**: Support stable blood sugar levels by avoiding processed sugars and refined carbohydrates.

5. Enhanced Mental Clarity and Mood

- **Mood Stabilization**: Improve mood and cognitive function by providing essential nutrients and reducing inflammatory foods.
- **Stress Reduction**: Implement dietary changes that help manage stress and anxiety levels.

6. Support for Immune Function

- **Nutrient-Rich Foods**: Include foods high in vitamins, minerals, and antioxidants to strengthen the immune system.

- **Hydration**: Emphasize the importance of hydration to support overall health and detoxification processes.

7. Development of Healthy Habits

- **Mindful Eating**: Encourage mindful eating practices that promote awareness of food choices and portion sizes.
- **Sustainable Changes**: Aim for long-term dietary changes rather than quick fixes, fostering a healthier lifestyle.

8. Improvement in Skin Health

- **Clear Skin**: Promote skin health by eliminating foods that may contribute to acne or other skin issues and focusing on hydrating, nutrient-rich foods.

9. Support for Healthy Aging

- **Anti-Aging Benefits**: Incorporate antioxidant-rich foods that may help reduce the signs of aging and promote overall longevity.

10. Customized Approach

- **Individual Needs**: Tailor the detox approach to meet individual dietary preferences, restrictions, and health goals.

By focusing on these goals, dietary detox can contribute to a healthier lifestyle and improved overall well-being.

Common components of detox diets typically focus on whole, nutrient-dense foods while eliminating processed foods and potential toxins. Here are key components often found in detox diets:

1. Whole Foods

- **Fruits and Vegetables**: Emphasize a variety of fresh, organic fruits and vegetables for their vitamins, minerals, and antioxidants.
- **Whole Grains**: Include whole grains like quinoa, brown rice, and oats for fiber and sustained energy.

2. Hydration

- **Water**: Encourage increased water intake to support hydration and flush out toxins.
- **Herbal Teas**: Include herbal teas (e.g., dandelion, ginger, green tea) that may support detoxification and digestion.

3. Lean Proteins

- **Sources**: Incorporate lean proteins like chicken, turkey, fish, tofu, and legumes to support muscle health and satiety.

4. Healthy Fats

- **Sources**: Include healthy fats from sources like avocados, nuts, seeds, and olive oil to promote heart health and nutrient absorption.

5. Fiber-Rich Foods

- **Role**: High-fiber foods help support digestion and regular bowel movements, aiding in the elimination of waste.

6. Probiotics

- **Sources**: Include fermented foods like yogurt, kefir, sauerkraut, and kimchi to support gut health and improve digestion.

7. Elimination of Processed Foods

- **Avoid**: Remove refined sugars, artificial additives, and highly processed foods to reduce toxin intake.

8. Limited Caffeine and Alcohol

- **Caffeine**: Reduce or eliminate caffeine to support overall detoxification and minimize dehydration.
- **Alcohol**: Avoid alcohol to give the liver a break and support recovery.

9. Mindful Eating

- **Practice**: Encourage mindful eating habits, focusing on portion control and awareness of hunger cues.

10. Temporary Elimination of Certain Foods

- **Common Eliminations**: Some detox diets may temporarily eliminate dairy, gluten, and high-sugar foods to assess sensitivities or reduce inflammation.

These components aim to enhance overall health, support the body's natural detoxification processes, and foster healthier eating habits.

Here are some popular detox diets that many people follow to promote health and well-being:

1. Juice Cleanse

- **Overview**: Involves consuming only fruit and vegetable juices for a set period, usually ranging from 1 to 7 days.
- **Purpose**: Aims to flood the body with nutrients while allowing the digestive system to rest.
- **Components**: Freshly pressed juices, typically made from greens, citrus fruits, and other vegetables.

2. Whole30

- **Overview**: A 30-day program that eliminates sugar, grains, dairy, legumes, and processed foods.
- **Purpose**: Focuses on whole, unprocessed foods to reset eating habits and identify food sensitivities.
- **Components**: Whole foods like fruits, vegetables, meats, seafood, nuts, and healthy fats.

3. Mediterranean Diet

- **Overview**: A long-term dietary pattern based on traditional foods from countries bordering the Mediterranean Sea.

- **Purpose**: Promotes heart health and overall well-being, with an emphasis on healthy fats and whole foods.
- **Components**: Olive oil, fish, whole grains, fruits, vegetables, nuts, and moderate wine consumption.

4. The 21-Day Detox

- **Overview**: A structured program that often includes meal plans and recipes to guide food choices for three weeks.
- **Purpose**: To eliminate toxins from the diet while focusing on nutrient-rich foods.
- **Components**: Whole foods, smoothies, salads, lean proteins, and elimination of sugar and processed foods.

5. Clean Eating

- **Overview**: Focuses on eating whole, minimally processed foods while avoiding artificial ingredients and added sugars.
- **Purpose**: Aims for overall health improvement and sustainable eating habits.
- **Components**: Fruits, vegetables, whole grains, lean proteins, and healthy fats, while avoiding refined and processed foods.

6. Master Cleanse (Lemon Detox)

- **Overview**: A liquid detox diet consisting of a mixture of water, lemon juice, maple syrup, and cayenne pepper.
- **Purpose**: Claims to detoxify the body and promote weight loss; typically lasts 10 days or more.
- **Components**: Only the lemon drink; no solid foods are consumed during the cleanse.

7. Vegan Detox

- **Overview**: A short-term vegan diet focusing on plant-based foods to promote health and detoxification.
- **Purpose**: Eliminates animal products and emphasizes nutrient-dense plant foods.

- **Components**: Fruits, vegetables, whole grains, nuts, seeds, and legumes.

Each of these diets has its own approach and intended benefits, so it's essential to choose one that aligns with your health goals and lifestyle.

Dietary detoxes can offer several potential benefits, especially when approached thoughtfully and as part of a broader health strategy. Here are some common benefits:

1. Increased Nutrient Intake

- **Focus on Whole Foods**: Emphasizes consumption of fruits, vegetables, and whole grains, leading to improved vitamin and mineral intake.

2. Improved Digestion

- **Gut Health**: A dietary detox often includes fiber-rich foods and probiotics, which can promote better digestion and a healthier gut microbiome.

3. Enhanced Energy Levels

- **Stable Blood Sugar**: By eliminating refined sugars and processed foods, many experience more stable energy levels and reduced fatigue.

4. Weight Management

- **Healthy Habits**: Detox diets can encourage healthier eating patterns, potentially leading to weight loss or maintenance.

5. Reduced Inflammation

- **Anti-Inflammatory Foods**: Many detox diets focus on anti-inflammatory foods, which may help reduce chronic inflammation in the body.

6. Improved Skin Health

- **Clearer Skin**: A diet rich in antioxidants and hydration can lead to improvements in skin appearance and health.

7. Enhanced Mental Clarity and Mood

- **Mood Stabilization**: Some individuals report improved focus and mood stability after eliminating processed foods and sugars.

8. Resetting Eating Habits

- **Mindful Eating**: A detox can serve as a reset, helping individuals become more aware of their food choices and develop healthier habits.

9. Support for Liver Function

- **Detoxification Support**: Emphasizing foods that support liver health can enhance the body's natural detoxification processes.

10. Increased Hydration

- **Water and Herbal Teas**: Encourages higher fluid intake, which is essential for overall health and detoxification.

11. Better Sleep

- **Improved Sleep Quality**: Some individuals experience better sleep as a result of dietary changes and reduced consumption of stimulants.

While these benefits can be appealing, it's essential to approach dietary detoxes with realistic expectations and consult healthcare professionals when necessary.

Dietary detoxes can offer several potential benefits, especially when approached thoughtfully and as part of a broader health strategy. Here are some common benefits:

1. Increased Nutrient Intake

- **Focus on Whole Foods**: Emphasizes consumption of fruits, vegetables, and whole grains, leading to improved vitamin and mineral intake.

2. Improved Digestion

- **Gut Health**: A dietary detox often includes fiber-rich foods and probiotics, which can promote better digestion and a healthier gut microbiome.

3. Enhanced Energy Levels

- **Stable Blood Sugar**: By eliminating refined sugars and processed foods, many experience more stable energy levels and reduced fatigue.

4. Weight Management

- **Healthy Habits**: Detox diets can encourage healthier eating patterns, potentially leading to weight loss or maintenance.

5. Reduced Inflammation

- **Anti-Inflammatory Foods**: Many detox diets focus on anti-inflammatory foods, which may help reduce chronic inflammation in the body.

6. Improved Skin Health

- **Clearer Skin**: A diet rich in antioxidants and hydration can lead to improvements in skin appearance and health.

7. Enhanced Mental Clarity and Mood

- **Mood Stabilization**: Some individuals report improved focus and mood stability after eliminating processed foods and sugars.

8. Resetting Eating Habits

- **Mindful Eating**: A detox can serve as a reset, helping individuals become more aware of their food choices and develop healthier habits.

9. Support for Liver Function

- **Detoxification Support**: Emphasizing foods that support liver health can enhance the body's natural detoxification processes.

10. Increased Hydration

- **Water and Herbal Teas**: Encourages higher fluid intake, which is essential for overall health and detoxification.

11. Better Sleep

- **Improved Sleep Quality**: Some individuals experience better sleep as a result of dietary changes and reduced consumption of stimulants.

While these benefits can be appealing, it's essential to approach dietary detoxes with realistic expectations and consult healthcare professionals when necessary.

While dietary detoxes can offer benefits, there are also potential risks and considerations to keep in mind:

1. Nutritional Deficiencies

- **Limited Food Variety**: Some detox diets may restrict food groups, leading to deficiencies in essential nutrients (vitamins, minerals, protein, healthy fats).

2. Temporary Weight Loss

- **Fluid Loss**: Initial weight loss may be primarily due to water loss rather than fat loss, which can be quickly regained after returning to regular eating.

3. Disordered Eating Patterns

- **Unhealthy Mindset**: Strict detox diets can trigger or exacerbate disordered eating behaviors or an unhealthy relationship with food.

4. Low Energy Levels

- **Fatigue**: Caloric restriction or elimination of food groups may lead to decreased energy levels and fatigue, affecting daily activities.

5. Gastrointestinal Issues

- **Digestive Discomfort**: Increased fiber intake or drastic dietary changes may cause bloating, gas, or digestive upset, especially if not gradually introduced.

6. Withdrawal Symptoms

- **Sugar and Caffeine**: Eliminating sugar or caffeine may lead to withdrawal symptoms such as headaches, irritability, and mood swings.

7. Medical Conditions

- **Pre-existing Conditions**: Individuals with certain health conditions (e.g., diabetes, eating disorders) should consult a healthcare provider before starting a detox diet.

8. Short-term Focus

- **Unsustainable Practices**: Many detox diets are not sustainable long-term, leading to a cycle of yo-yo dieting and potential weight regain.

9. Emotional Impact

- **Social and Emotional Effects**: Restrictive diets can lead to feelings of deprivation or social isolation, particularly in social situations involving food.

10. Misleading Claims

- **Detox Myths**: Be cautious of detox diets that promise rapid weight loss or miracle cures, as these claims are often exaggerated or unfounded.

Recommendations for Safe Detox

- **Consult a Professional**: Speak with a healthcare provider or registered dietitian before starting any detox diet, especially if you have underlying health conditions.
- **Focus on Balance**: Aim for a balanced approach that includes a variety of whole foods rather than extreme restrictions.
- **Listen to Your Body**: Pay attention to how your body responds to dietary changes and adjust accordingly.

By considering these risks and adopting a mindful approach, individuals can make informed decisions about dietary detoxes.

A balanced approach to detox focuses on promoting overall health without extreme restrictions or drastic changes. Here are key principles for a balanced detox:

1. Gradual Changes

- **Ease into Detox**: Make gradual dietary changes rather than abrupt shifts. Start by incorporating more whole foods and reducing processed foods over time.

2. Focus on Whole Foods

- **Emphasize Nutrient-Dense Options**: Prioritize fruits, vegetables, whole grains, lean proteins, and healthy fats. These foods provide essential nutrients and support overall health.

3. Stay Hydrated

- **Increase Water Intake**: Aim for adequate hydration through water and herbal teas. Proper hydration supports digestion and detoxification processes.

4. Mindful Eating

- **Practice Awareness**: Pay attention to hunger cues and eat slowly. This encourages a better relationship with food and helps prevent overeating.

5. Limit Processed Foods

- **Reduce Refined Sugars and Additives**: Minimize intake of processed foods, refined sugars, and artificial additives. Focus on cooking at home using fresh ingredients.

6. Listen to Your Body

- **Individual Needs**: Pay attention to how different foods affect your body. Adjust your diet based on personal preferences and any sensitivities.

7. Include Physical Activity

- **Regular Exercise**: Incorporate physical activity that you enjoy, such as walking, yoga, or dancing. Exercise supports detoxification and overall well-being.

8. Incorporate Mind-Body Practices

- **Stress Management**: Use techniques like meditation, deep breathing, or yoga to reduce stress, which can negatively impact health.

9. Set Realistic Goals

- **Sustainable Changes**: Focus on long-term health rather than quick fixes. Set achievable goals for gradual improvement in dietary habits.

10. Seek Professional Guidance

- **Consult Experts**: Work with a registered dietitian or healthcare professional for personalized advice and to ensure nutritional adequacy during detox.

By adopting this balanced approach, you can support your body's natural detoxification processes while promoting sustainable health practices.

The goals of environmental detox focus on reducing exposure to harmful substances in one's surroundings and promoting overall health and well-being. Here are key objectives:

1. Reduce Toxic Exposure

- **Eliminate Harmful Chemicals**: Aim to minimize exposure to toxins from household products, pollutants, and chemicals in food and personal care items.

2. Improve Indoor Air Quality

- **Ventilation and Purification**: Enhance indoor air quality by increasing ventilation, using air purifiers, and incorporating plants that can help filter pollutants.

3. Promote Safe Personal Care Products

- **Natural Alternatives**: Choose personal care and cleaning products that are free from harmful chemicals, such as parabens, phthalates, and synthetic fragrances.

4. Enhance Water Quality

- **Water Filtration**: Use water filtration systems to reduce contaminants and improve the quality of drinking and cooking water.

5. Support Sustainable Practices

- **Reduce Waste**: Adopt practices that minimize waste, such as recycling and composting, to lessen environmental impact.

6. Encourage Natural Cleaning Solutions

- **DIY Products**: Use natural cleaning solutions (e.g., vinegar, baking soda) to clean your home without harsh chemicals.

7. Increase Awareness of Food Sources

- **Organic and Local Foods**: Support local farmers and choose organic foods to reduce exposure to pesticides and additives.

8. Foster Healthy Habits

- **Lifestyle Changes**: Promote healthier lifestyle choices that reduce reliance on products with harmful ingredients (e.g., smoking cessation, reduced use of plastics).

9. Cultivate Mindfulness and Stress Reduction

- **Stress Management**: Engage in practices such as mindfulness and meditation to enhance mental well-being and cope with environmental stressors.

10. Community Engagement

- **Advocate for Change**: Get involved in community efforts to reduce environmental toxins and promote policies that protect public health.

By focusing on these goals, individuals can create a healthier living environment and reduce the negative impacts of environmental toxins on their health.

Common environmental toxins can be found in various aspects of daily life, including air, water, soil, and consumer products. Here are some of the most prevalent environmental toxins:

1. Air Pollutants

- **Particulate Matter (PM)**: Tiny particles from vehicle emissions, industrial processes, and natural sources that can affect respiratory health.
- **Volatile Organic Compounds (VOCs)**: Emitted from paints, cleaning supplies, and building materials; can contribute to indoor air pollution.
- **Nitrogen Dioxide (NO2)**: From combustion processes (e.g., vehicles, heating) and can lead to respiratory issues.

2. Heavy Metals

- **Lead**: Found in old paint, plumbing, and contaminated soil; can affect neurological development.
- **Mercury**: Present in some fish, dental amalgams, and industrial discharges; harmful to the nervous system.
- **Cadmium**: Found in batteries, certain fertilizers, and contaminated food/water; can damage kidneys and bones.

3. Pesticides

- **Herbicides and Insecticides**: Chemicals used in agriculture and home gardening that can have harmful effects on human health and the environment.

4. Chemicals in Consumer Products

- **Phthalates**: Found in plastics and personal care products; linked to hormonal disruptions.
- **BPA (Bisphenol A)**: Used in plastics and can leach into food and beverages; associated with endocrine disruption.

5. Water Contaminants

- **Chlorine and Chloramines**: Used in water treatment but can form harmful byproducts that may be carcinogenic.
- **Fluoride**: Added to drinking water for dental health, but excessive exposure can lead to health issues.

6. Mold and Mildew

- **Indoor Fungi**: Can produce mycotoxins that affect respiratory health and immune function, especially in damp environments.

7. Asbestos

- **Building Material**: Once used for insulation and fireproofing, inhaling asbestos fibers can lead to serious lung diseases.

8. Radon

- **Natural Gas**: A colorless, odorless gas that can accumulate in homes, especially in basements, and is a known carcinogen.

9. Industrial Chemicals

- **PCBs (Polychlorinated Biphenyls)**: Used in electrical equipment; persistent in the environment and harmful to health.
- **Dioxins**: Byproducts of industrial processes that can accumulate in the food chain and pose health risks.

10. Endocrine Disruptors

- **Chemicals that Interfere with Hormones**: Found in various products and can lead to reproductive and developmental issues.

Reducing exposure to these toxins involves making informed choices about products, improving indoor air quality, and advocating for environmental policies.

Here are effective strategies for environmental detox that can help reduce exposure to harmful toxins and promote a healthier living environment:

1. Improve Indoor Air Quality

- **Ventilation**: Regularly open windows and use exhaust fans to improve air circulation.

- **Air Purifiers**: Invest in HEPA air purifiers to filter out airborne pollutants and allergens.
- **Houseplants**: Incorporate indoor plants known for their air-purifying properties (e.g., spider plants, peace lilies).

2. Reduce Chemical Exposure

- **Natural Cleaning Products**: Use non-toxic or homemade cleaning solutions (e.g., vinegar, baking soda) instead of commercial cleaners.
- **Personal Care Products**: Choose personal care items free from harmful chemicals, such as parabens and phthalates. Look for "clean" or organic labels.
- **Minimize Plastics**: Reduce the use of plastic containers, especially for food storage; opt for glass or stainless steel alternatives.

3. Ensure Water Quality

- **Water Filtration**: Use water filters to remove contaminants from drinking water. Consider reverse osmosis systems for comprehensive purification.
- **Check for Lead**: If in an older home, test for lead in plumbing and consider replacing lead pipes or using water filters designed to remove lead.

4. Minimize Pesticide Use

- **Organic Gardening**: If gardening, use organic methods and natural pest control instead of synthetic pesticides.
- **Wash Produce**: Thoroughly wash fruits and vegetables to reduce pesticide residues.

5. Declutter and Organize

- **Reduce Clutter**: Minimize clutter in your home to improve air circulation and reduce dust accumulation, which can harbor toxins.
- **Proper Storage**: Store chemicals and cleaning supplies securely and out of reach of children and pets.

6. Be Mindful of Food Sources

- **Choose Organic**: When possible, select organic produce to reduce exposure to pesticides and synthetic fertilizers.
- **Support Local**: Buy food from local farmers or farmers' markets to minimize the carbon footprint and support sustainable practices.

7. Practice Sustainable Living

- **Reduce Waste**: Compost organic waste and recycle materials to minimize landfill contributions.
- **Conserve Energy**: Use energy-efficient appliances and light bulbs to reduce energy consumption and associated pollutants.

8. Educate and Advocate

- **Stay Informed**: Keep up with research and news on environmental toxins and health impacts.
- **Community Involvement**: Participate in community clean-up efforts and advocate for policies that promote environmental health.

9. Limit Exposure to Heavy Metals

- **Avoid Certain Fish**: Be cautious with fish known to have high mercury levels (e.g., swordfish, shark).
- **Check for Lead**: If you live in an older home, check for lead-based paint and have it professionally removed if necessary.

10. Stress Management

- **Mindfulness Practices**: Engage in activities like yoga, meditation, and deep breathing to reduce stress, which can negatively impact health.

By implementing these strategies, you can create a healthier environment for yourself and your family while reducing exposure to harmful toxins.

Here are additional tips for environmental detox that can further enhance your efforts to reduce exposure to toxins and promote a healthier living space:

1. Regular Cleaning

- **Dust and Vacuum**: Clean regularly to reduce dust accumulation, which can harbor allergens and toxins. Use a vacuum with a HEPA filter.
- **Wash Bedding and Curtains**: Regularly wash bedding, curtains, and upholstery to remove dust mites and allergens.

2. Choose Natural Fabrics

- **Organic Textiles**: Opt for organic cotton, linen, or wool for bedding and clothing to avoid pesticides and harmful chemicals found in conventional fabrics.

3. Avoid Artificial Fragrances

- **Fragrance-Free Products**: Choose cleaning and personal care products that are fragrance-free or use essential oils for natural scents.

4. Limit Electromagnetic Field (EMF) Exposure

- **Reduce Screen Time**: Limit prolonged exposure to screens and consider using EMF shielding products if concerned about exposure.
- **Distance Devices**: Keep electronic devices at a distance when not in use, especially while sleeping.

5. Opt for Non-Toxic Cookware

- **Choose Safe Materials**: Use cookware made of stainless steel, cast iron, or glass instead of non-stick coatings that can release harmful chemicals at high temperatures.

6. Stay Informed About Environmental Issues

- **Follow Local Policies**: Stay updated on local environmental regulations and initiatives that impact your community's health and safety.

7. Practice Sustainable Transportation

- **Walk or Bike**: Use walking, biking, or public transportation to reduce carbon emissions and air pollution.
- **Carpool**: Share rides when possible to decrease the number of vehicles on the road.

8. Reduce Use of Personal Care Products

- **Simplify Routine**: Streamline your personal care routine to essential products to reduce exposure to multiple chemicals.

9. Check Home for Radon

- **Test for Radon**: Use radon testing kits to check your home's radon levels, especially in basements, and take action if levels are high.

10. Educate Others

- **Share Knowledge**: Educate family and friends about environmental toxins and sustainable practices to foster a community-focused approach to health.

Incorporating these tips can help create a healthier living environment and minimize exposure to harmful substances.

The benefits of environmental detox focus on reducing exposure to harmful toxins and enhancing overall health and well-being. Here are some key advantages:

1. Improved Health

- **Reduced Illness Risk**: Lower exposure to toxins can decrease the risk of chronic diseases, including respiratory issues, cardiovascular problems, and certain cancers.

2. Enhanced Immune Function

- **Stronger Immunity**: Reducing toxin exposure can support a healthier immune system, making it more effective at fighting off illnesses.

3. Better Respiratory Health

- **Cleaner Air**: Improving indoor air quality can lead to fewer respiratory issues, such as asthma and allergies, and promote easier breathing.

4. Increased Energy Levels

- **Less Toxic Load**: A cleaner environment can lead to improved energy levels, reducing fatigue and enhancing overall vitality.

5. Mental Clarity and Mood Improvement

- **Cognitive Benefits**: Reducing exposure to environmental toxins can positively impact brain health, leading to improved focus, memory, and mood.

6. Healthier Living Spaces

- **Safer Home Environment**: Detoxifying your environment can create a safer and more pleasant living space, reducing clutter and promoting well-being.

7. Sustainable Practices

- **Environmental Impact**: Adopting detox strategies often aligns with sustainable living practices, contributing to a healthier planet.

8. Long-term Wellness

- **Preventive Health**: Taking steps to detox the environment can promote long-term health and well-being, reducing the likelihood of toxin-related health issues.

9. Enhanced Sleep Quality

- **Better Sleep Environment**: A cleaner, less toxic living space can lead to improved sleep quality, supporting overall health and recovery.

10. Community Awareness

- **Increased Engagement**: Participating in environmental detox efforts can raise awareness in your community, encouraging collective action for better health.

By focusing on these benefits, individuals can create a healthier and more sustainable lifestyle that enhances both personal well-being and environmental health.

The goals of a digital detox focus on reducing screen time and the overall impact of digital devices on mental and physical well-being. Here are key objectives:

1. Reduce Screen Time

- **Limit Usage**: Decrease the amount of time spent on devices to foster healthier habits and relationships.

2. Improve Mental Health

- **Reduce Stress and Anxiety**: Minimize exposure to social media and constant notifications, which can contribute to stress and anxiety.

3. Enhance Focus and Productivity

- **Boost Concentration**: Limit distractions from devices to improve focus and productivity in work and daily activities.

4. Foster Real-Life Connections

- **Strengthen Relationships**: Encourage face-to-face interactions with friends and family, enhancing social bonds and emotional support.

5. Improve Sleep Quality

- **Reduce Blue Light Exposure**: Limit screen use before bedtime to improve sleep quality and regulate sleep patterns.

6. Increase Mindfulness

- **Promote Presence**: Encourage mindfulness and being present in the moment by reducing distractions from digital devices.

7. Reclaim Time

- **Rediscover Hobbies**: Free up time to engage in offline activities, hobbies, and interests that may have been neglected.

8. Encourage Outdoor Activity

- **Promote Physical Activity**: Inspire more time spent outdoors, which can enhance physical health and overall well-being.

9. Evaluate Digital Habits

- **Reflect on Usage**: Gain awareness of digital habits and identify patterns that may be unhealthy or unproductive.

10. Cultivate Digital Boundaries

- **Set Healthy Limits**: Establish boundaries for device use to create a healthier relationship with technology in the long term.

By focusing on these goals, individuals can enhance their quality of life and create a more balanced relationship with technology.

Here are some signs that you might benefit from a digital detox:

1. Constant Distraction

- **Difficulty Focusing**: Struggling to concentrate on tasks due to frequent interruptions from notifications or the urge to check devices.

2. Increased Anxiety or Stress

- **Feeling Overwhelmed**: Experiencing anxiety related to social media, emails, or online interactions, leading to heightened stress levels.

3. Sleep Disturbances

- **Trouble Sleeping**: Difficulty falling asleep or staying asleep, often due to screen time before bed or the influence of digital devices on sleep patterns.

4. Reduced Face-to-Face Interaction

- **Social Isolation**: Spending more time interacting online than in person, leading to feelings of loneliness or disconnection from others.

5. Decreased Productivity

- **Procrastination**: Using devices as a way to procrastinate or distract from important tasks, impacting overall productivity.

6. Physical Symptoms

- **Eye Strain and Fatigue**: Experiencing symptoms like headaches, eye strain, or fatigue related to prolonged screen use.

7. Impaired Relationships

- **Neglected Connections**: Noticing a decline in the quality of personal relationships due to excessive time spent online or on devices.

8. Compulsive Behavior

- **Constant Checking**: Feeling the need to check notifications or social media repeatedly, even when not necessary.

9. Lack of Mindfulness

- **Living in the Digital World**: Feeling disconnected from the present moment and more focused on online content than real-life experiences.

10. Feeling Unfulfilled

- **Discontent with Online Engagement**: Experiencing dissatisfaction with time spent online, questioning its value or impact on personal happiness.

If you identify with several of these signs, a digital detox may help improve your mental well-being and overall quality of life.

Here are steps for a successful digital detox:

1. Set Clear Goals

- **Define Objectives**: Determine why you want to detox (e.g., reduce stress, improve sleep, enhance focus) and set specific, achievable goals.

2. Create a Detox Plan

- **Choose Duration**: Decide how long you'll detox (e.g., a weekend, a week, or longer).
- **Identify Devices**: List the devices and platforms you want to limit (e.g., smartphones, social media, gaming).

3. Inform Others

- **Communicate Your Intentions**: Let friends, family, and colleagues know about your detox to manage expectations and encourage support.

4. Set Boundaries

- **Limit Usage**: Establish specific times for device use or create tech-free zones (e.g., during meals or in the bedroom).
- **Schedule Breaks**: Plan regular breaks from screens throughout the day.

5. Replace Digital Activities

- **Engage in Offline Hobbies**: Find alternative activities like reading, exercising, cooking, or spending time outdoors to fill the time previously spent online.

6. Unsubscribe and Declutter

- **Reduce Notifications**: Unsubscribe from unnecessary emails and turn off non-essential notifications to minimize distractions.
- **Clean Up Your Devices**: Organize apps and files to create a more streamlined digital experience.

7. Practice Mindfulness

- **Stay Present**: Use mindfulness techniques, such as meditation or deep breathing, to cultivate awareness and reduce the urge to check devices.

8. Evaluate Progress

- **Reflect Regularly**: Take time to assess how the detox is impacting your mood, focus, and overall well-being.

9. Gradual Reintroduction

- **Ease Back In**: After the detox period, gradually reintroduce technology while maintaining boundaries to avoid reverting to old habits.

10. Make It a Habit

- **Ongoing Detox**: Consider scheduling regular digital detox periods in the future to maintain balance and mindfulness in your relationship with technology.

By following these steps, you can successfully navigate a digital detox and reap the benefits of a healthier balance with technology.

Here are some tips for maintaining a digital detox after your initial period:

1. Establish Tech-Free Zones

- **Designate Areas**: Create spaces in your home (like the bedroom or dining area) where devices are not allowed to encourage real-life interactions.

2. Set Specific Times for Device Use

- **Scheduled Check-Ins**: Allocate specific times during the day to check emails or social media, limiting spontaneous usage.

3. Use Apps Mindfully

- **Limit Notifications**: Turn off non-essential notifications to reduce distractions and interruptions throughout the day.

4. Replace Digital Activities with Offline Options

- **Engage in Hobbies**: Find offline hobbies (like reading, crafting, or exercising) to fill time previously spent online and enhance your well-being.

5. Practice Mindfulness

- **Mindful Tech Use**: Be intentional about how and when you use technology. Before reaching for your device, ask yourself if it's necessary.

6. Keep a Journal

- **Reflect on Your Experience**: Regularly jot down thoughts about your digital habits and how you feel when you limit screen time.

7. Prioritize Face-to-Face Interactions

- **Schedule In-Person Time**: Make plans with friends and family to connect in person, fostering deeper relationships and reducing reliance on digital communication.

8. Regular Digital Detoxes

- **Plan Short Breaks**: Consider periodic digital detoxes to reset your habits and maintain a healthy relationship with technology.

9. Educate Yourself

- **Stay Informed**: Read about the effects of excessive screen time on mental and physical health to reinforce your commitment to digital well-being.

10. Share Your Journey

- **Encourage Others**: Share your experiences with friends and family, inspiring them to consider their digital habits and possibly join you in a digital detox.

By integrating these tips into your routine, you can maintain a balanced approach to technology use and continue enjoying the benefits of a digital detox.

Here are the benefits of a digital detox:

1. Reduced Stress and Anxiety

- **Less Digital Overload**: Decreased exposure to social media and constant notifications can lower stress levels and anxiety.

2. Improved Mental Clarity

- **Enhanced Focus**: Less distraction from screens can lead to better concentration and productivity.

3. Better Sleep Quality

- **Regulated Sleep Patterns**: Reducing screen time, especially before bed, can improve sleep quality and duration.

4. Strengthened Relationships

- **Increased Face-to-Face Interaction**: More time spent offline fosters deeper connections with family and friends.

5. Enhanced Creativity

- **More Mental Space**: Stepping away from screens can open up time for creative thinking and exploration of new interests.

6. Greater Mindfulness

- **Present Moment Awareness**: A digital detox encourages mindfulness and being present in the moment, leading to a more fulfilling life.

7. Better Physical Health

- **Increased Activity**: With less time on devices, there's more opportunity for physical activities, contributing to overall health.

8. Improved Mood

- **Less Comparison and FOMO**: Reducing exposure to social media can decrease feelings of inadequacy and fear of missing out (FOMO), leading to a more positive outlook.

9. Enhanced Productivity

- **Fewer Distractions**: Less screen time can result in greater efficiency and output in both personal and professional tasks.

10. Greater Awareness of Digital Habits

- **Informed Choices**: A digital detox encourages reflection on how technology impacts your life, promoting healthier usage patterns moving forward.

By engaging in a digital detox, you can enjoy these benefits, leading to a more balanced and fulfilling life.

Here are common challenges faced during a digital detox and potential solutions:

1. Withdrawal Symptoms

Challenge: Feelings of anxiety or restlessness when disconnected from devices.

- **Solution**: Gradually reduce screen time instead of an abrupt detox. Replace digital activities with engaging offline hobbies to ease the transition.

2. Social Pressure

Challenge: Fear of missing out (FOMO) or feeling disconnected from friends and social circles.

- **Solution**: Communicate your detox goals with friends and family. Schedule in-person meet-ups or share experiences offline to maintain connections.

3. Work Obligations

Challenge: The need to stay connected for professional reasons can make detoxing difficult.

- **Solution**: Set specific times for checking work emails and messages, allowing you to maintain work responsibilities while still detoxing.

4. Boredom

Challenge: Feeling bored without digital distractions.

- **Solution**: Create a list of offline activities you enjoy (reading, exercising, crafting) and make a commitment to engage in them during your detox.

5. Habitual Use

Challenge: Difficulty breaking ingrained habits of reaching for devices automatically.

- **Solution**: Identify triggers that lead to device use and develop alternative responses (e.g., take a walk or do a quick workout instead).

6. Information Overload

Challenge: Missing out on important updates or news while detoxing.

- **Solution**: Schedule specific times to catch up on essential news and information after your detox period, ensuring you stay informed without constant checking.

7. Family and Household Dynamics

Challenge: Other household members may not be on board with a digital detox, leading to distractions.

- **Solution**: Involve family members in the detox process, setting shared tech-free times or activities that everyone can enjoy together.

8. Lack of Motivation

Challenge: Finding it hard to stay motivated throughout the detox.

- **Solution:** Set specific, measurable goals for your detox, and track your progress. Celebrate small wins to keep your motivation high.

By anticipating these challenges and implementing solutions, you can have a more successful and rewarding digital detox experience.

The goals of an emotional and mental detox focus on promoting mental well-being and emotional clarity. Here are key objectives:

1. Reduce Mental Clutter

- **Clear Thought Processes:** Eliminate negative thoughts and distractions, leading to improved focus and clarity.

2. Enhance Emotional Awareness

- **Understand Emotions:** Increase awareness of your feelings, helping you identify and process them more effectively.

3. Improve Stress Management

- **Develop Coping Strategies:** Learn techniques to manage stress and anxiety, fostering resilience in challenging situations.

4. Cultivate Mindfulness

- **Be Present:** Encourage mindfulness practices to stay grounded in the present moment, reducing overthinking and worry about the future.

5. Strengthen Self-Compassion

- **Promote Kindness to Self:** Foster a more compassionate attitude towards yourself, reducing self-criticism and enhancing self-esteem.

6. Build Healthy Boundaries

- **Protect Emotional Space**: Learn to establish boundaries in relationships and commitments, ensuring emotional well-being.

7. Foster Positive Relationships

- **Improve Connections**: Enhance communication skills and emotional intelligence to strengthen existing relationships and build new ones.

8. Increase Resilience

- **Adapt to Challenges**: Develop a more resilient mindset, enabling you to bounce back from setbacks and navigate difficulties with greater ease.

9. Encourage Self-Reflection

- **Assess Personal Growth**: Regularly reflect on your emotions and mental state, identifying patterns and areas for growth.

10. Promote Overall Well-Being

- **Enhance Life Satisfaction**: Focus on improving mental health and emotional stability, leading to a more fulfilling and balanced life.

By pursuing these goals, individuals can achieve greater emotional balance and mental clarity, leading to improved overall well-being.

Here are signs that you might benefit from an emotional and mental detox:

1. Overwhelm and Stress

- **Constant Feeling of Being Overloaded**: Experiencing chronic stress or feeling overwhelmed by daily responsibilities and emotions.

2. Increased Anxiety or Irritability

- **Frequent Mood Swings**: Noticing heightened anxiety, irritability, or frustration that feels disproportionate to the situation.

3. Difficulty Concentrating

- **Struggling to Focus**: Having trouble concentrating or making decisions due to mental clutter and distractions.

4. Emotional Exhaustion

- **Feeling Drained**: Experiencing emotional fatigue, feeling drained after social interactions, or lacking enthusiasm for activities you usually enjoy.

5. Negative Thought Patterns

- **Persistent Negative Thinking**: Engaging in repetitive negative thoughts or self-criticism, impacting self-esteem and overall outlook.

6. Withdrawal from Social Interactions

- **Isolation**: Withdrawing from friends and family or feeling disconnected from others, leading to increased loneliness.

7. Difficulty Managing Emotions

- **Emotional Dysregulation**: Struggling to manage your emotions, leading to outbursts or feeling numb.

8. Lack of Motivation

- **Diminished Drive**: Experiencing a lack of motivation or interest in activities, work, or personal goals.

9. Trouble Sleeping

- **Insomnia or Poor Sleep Quality**: Experiencing sleep disturbances, such as difficulty falling asleep or frequent waking, often due to racing thoughts.

10. Feeling Stuck

- **Lack of Direction**: Sensing stagnation in personal growth or feeling stuck in negative patterns without clarity on how to move forward.

If you identify with several of these signs, an emotional and mental detox may help you regain balance and enhance your well-being.

Here are steps for an effective emotional and mental detox:

1. Set Intentions

- **Define Your Goals**: Clarify what you hope to achieve, such as reducing stress, enhancing emotional awareness, or improving mental clarity.

2. Create a Safe Space

- **Find a Quiet Environment**: Designate a calming space where you can reflect, meditate, or journal without distractions.

3. Practice Mindfulness and Meditation

- **Incorporate Mindfulness**: Engage in mindfulness exercises or meditation to stay present and cultivate awareness of your thoughts and feelings.

4. Journal Your Thoughts

- **Write Regularly**: Keep a journal to express your emotions, track patterns, and reflect on your experiences. This can provide clarity and insight.

5. Limit Negative Influences

- **Reduce Exposure**: Identify and limit contact with negative people or environments that drain your energy or provoke stress.

6. Establish Healthy Boundaries

- **Communicate Needs**: Learn to say no and establish boundaries in relationships and commitments to protect your emotional well-being.

7. Engage in Physical Activity

- **Exercise Regularly**: Incorporate physical activity into your routine, as exercise can boost mood and reduce stress.

8. Nourish Your Body

- **Eat Mindfully**: Focus on a balanced diet that supports mental health. Consider foods rich in omega-3s, antioxidants, and vitamins.

9. Connect with Nature

- **Spend Time Outdoors**: Spend time in nature to recharge and gain perspective, promoting relaxation and emotional balance.

10. Seek Support

- **Talk to Someone**: Consider discussing your feelings with a trusted friend, family member, or mental health professional for additional support.

11. Reflect and Adjust

- **Regular Check-Ins**: Periodically assess how you're feeling and what strategies are working. Be open to adjusting your approach as needed.

By following these steps, you can effectively detox emotionally and mentally, leading to greater clarity, balance, and well-being.

Here are additional strategies for an emotional and mental detox:

1. Digital Detox

- **Limit Screen Time**: Reduce time spent on social media and devices to decrease information overload and anxiety.

2. Practice Gratitude

- **Daily Gratitude Journaling**: Write down things you're grateful for each day to shift focus from negativity to positivity.

3. Engage in Creative Outlets

- **Explore Creativity**: Try activities like painting, writing, or music to express emotions and stimulate positive feelings.

4. Prioritize Sleep

- **Establish a Sleep Routine**: Create a consistent sleep schedule and bedtime routine to improve sleep quality and mental clarity.

5. Learn to Let Go

- **Release Negative Emotions**: Practice forgiveness and let go of grudges or past hurts that may be weighing you down.

6. Spend Time with Animals

- **Animal Interaction**: Spend time with pets or animals, as they can provide comfort, reduce stress, and promote emotional well-being.

7. Attend Workshops or Classes

- **Personal Development**: Participate in workshops or classes focused on emotional health, mindfulness, or self-improvement.

8. Volunteer or Help Others

- **Community Engagement**: Volunteering can provide a sense of purpose and connection, improving your mood and outlook.

9. Practice Breathing Exercises

- **Deep Breathing**: Use deep breathing techniques to calm your mind and body, reducing anxiety and promoting relaxation.

10. Seek Professional Help

- **Therapy or Counseling**: Consider talking to a therapist or counselor for guidance and support in navigating emotional challenges.

Implementing these strategies can further enhance your emotional and mental detox journey, leading to improved well-being and resilience.

Here are common challenges faced during an emotional and mental detox, along with potential solutions:

1. Resistance to Change

Challenge: Feeling uncomfortable or resistant to addressing emotions or breaking old habits.

- **Solution**: Start small by setting manageable goals and gradually introduce new practices, allowing yourself time to adjust.

2. Overwhelming Emotions

Challenge: Encountering strong emotions that are difficult to process or manage.

- **Solution**: Use grounding techniques, such as deep breathing or mindfulness, to stay present. Journaling can also help you articulate and process your feelings.

3. Distractions and Interruptions

Challenge: Difficulty finding quiet time due to external distractions or a busy schedule.

- **Solution**: Schedule dedicated time for your detox activities and communicate this to others, establishing boundaries to minimize interruptions.

4. Lack of Motivation

Challenge: Struggling to stay motivated throughout the detox process.

- **Solution**: Identify your "why" for detoxing, and track your progress. Celebrate small victories to maintain enthusiasm.

5. Fear of Confronting Emotions

Challenge: Avoiding the discomfort of facing unresolved feelings or past experiences.

- **Solution**: Consider seeking support from a therapist or counselor, who can provide a safe space to explore these emotions and guide you through the process.

6. Social Pressure

Challenge: Feeling pressured to engage in digital or social activities while detoxing.

- **Solution**: Communicate your intentions to friends and family. Surround yourself with supportive individuals who respect your detox goals.

7. Difficulty Maintaining Boundaries

Challenge: Struggling to establish or maintain boundaries with others.

- **Solution**: Practice assertive communication. Role-play scenarios with a trusted friend or write down what you want to express to build confidence.

8. Information Overload

Challenge: Feeling overwhelmed by the amount of information available on mental health and self-care.

- **Solution**: Focus on one or two strategies that resonate with you, rather than trying to implement everything at once. Simplify your approach.

9. Discomfort with Silence

Challenge: Finding it challenging to be in silence or solitude without distractions.

- **Solution**: Gradually increase time spent in silence, starting with short periods and gradually extending as you become more comfortable.

10. Difficulty Finding Support

Challenge: Feeling isolated in your detox journey.

- **Solution**: Look for local support groups, online communities, or workshops that focus on emotional well-being and mental health.

By anticipating these challenges and implementing practical solutions, you can enhance your emotional and mental detox experience, leading to greater clarity and well-being.

CONCLUSION

A full body detox can be beneficial for promoting overall health and well-being, but it's important to approach it with care. While many people report feeling more energetic and lighter after detoxing, the scientific evidence supporting the need for detox diets is limited.

Detoxing can encourage healthier eating habits, increased water intake, and mindfulness about food choices. However, extreme detox regimens can lead to nutritional deficiencies and other health issues.

In conclusion, if considering a detox, it's best to choose gentle, balanced methods that focus on whole foods, hydration, and lifestyle changes rather than restrictive diets. Always consult with a healthcare professional before starting any detox program to ensure it aligns with your individual health needs.